Like It Is

Like It Is

Francois Degraff

Library of Congress Control Number: 2010905389
ISBN: Hardcover   978-1-4500-8554-0
                Softcover   978-1-4500-8553-3
                Ebook   978-1-4500-8555-7

This book was printed in the United States of America.

To order additional copies of this book, contact:
Xlibris Corporation
1-888-795-4274
www.Xlibris.com
Orders@Xlibris.com
78341

Acknowledgments

I am indebted to my wife, Linda, who has devoted her life to put up with me during the years that we have been together, to my children Kathia and Cois who have spent their early years dealing with my grumpy attitude, and to my dog Nina who by her mischievousness never stops to tease me by fetching my socks wherever they may be and runs all around the house with them.

I am also indebted to America for allowing me to be in the land of the free and the brave, giving me the protection through freedom of speech telling it *Like It Is*!

Chapter 1

I chose this title not for the fun of it but to bring facts to the awareness of the people about what I have seen going on during my more than twenty years of experience while working in long-term care facilities.

It was heartache to see what had occurred in some of the facilities where I had worked—as the saying goes: when you see one, you have seen all—although there could be some exceptions.

The names used in *Like It Is* are fictional, to thwart any repercussion or predicaments in provisions of making decisions of which home is better than another, which could bring the extinction of some long-term care facilities.

What I am going to tell the people is the truth, because I was the eyewitness to these roguish practices and no one can contest it—the truth that I am going to tell will be hard to take but the public will eventually recognize it as true.

I came to Cleveland in the 1980s. I am a registered professional nurse. I liked the atmosphere, the calm, and quietude; I said to myself, *This is the place I want to be in until I go to my grave*. It was not without hardship at the beginning—to recall, I used to take a bus called the RTA every morning. Although I caught the bus at the same time, and saw the same faces, no one ever uttered a word to me, not even to say hello, the irony to that. It was a cold winter day. While riding the bus, I placed my hat, that I had got from New York for a dollar, on the seat beside me and when I turned my head to pick up my hat so that I could get off the bus my hat was gone. I missed my hat, a hat that had kept my head warm; I never experienced runny eyes or rhinorrhea—a one-dollar hat that I appreciated very much for the convenience it provided to me. Perhaps this clochard who took it did not know the importance and the history of this hat, wore it once, sold it for a fix, or kept it in his back pocket. This crook, who took my hat, never thought about me catching a cold and was not concerned that I had a family to provide for. He who steals a penny from the poor causes great discomfort to the poor, and will eventually steal from himself the opportunity, without end, to be a civilized and law-abiding person. I was very upset, thinking about this person who had stolen my shit; he would never get better in life. This individual's spirit was poor—he was the type of human being who makes the sorrow of the world.

While looking through the employment section of the local paper, I saw an ad for Whitecliff Manor, in search of registered nurses. The owner, a Jew, hired me right on the spot. I did not know the place was the pits. I started work. My first day of orientation was uneventful. I had a very tall nurse to show me the ropes. The conditions of the place did not bother me a bit. My second day of orientation was terrible. I punched in, reported to my floor for orientation, and was told by the night nurse that a nurse had called off, and the floor was mine. I took the key, counted the control drugs, and pushed the med cart to the floor. I hardly did any treatment, then signed out—I was pissed off. There was a so-called manager and LPN who was supposed to do the scheduling. As it was my second day, this nurse did not offer her help. I found out that this LPN had much power; she could hire and fire anyone without explanation. During my first week, I noted that every afternoon the light was off, the door locked, and even if an emergency occurred, there was no one in administration to contact although it was early afternoon. I was informed by the staff that the LPN and the so-called administrator stayed late and had a good time, almost every afternoon, enjoying the most euphoric time of their life.

Some of you would shake your head and say that this writer has balls. Let me tell you, "Yes, I do not only have balls but I carry the balls." Sometimes you just have to tell it *Like It Is*!

Chapter 2

At Whitecliff, the work was very hard due to the fact that the administrator did not provide enough help to care for the residents; at the end of the shift I would be exhausted. The administrator, greedy for money, did not want to lose a nurse's aide or to hire new ones for help in care. I recall here an incident about two nurse's aides at about 8:30 p.m. in the night shift. They were in the dining room exercising with the latest apparatus "the gut buster." The charge nurse wrote them up and sent the information to the administrator. He didn't take any corrective measures, patted them on the shoulder, and sent them back to the floor laughing. It was a kind of stressful situation for me to work under. I did work under stress for the short time that I was there. On my days off, not able to visit some new friends I remained in my room at the "Shangri-la," a name I hate, a place that I dreaded for the rest of my life. This place robbed me of the best souvenirs I had in my life—souvenirs that disappeared not through the result of a catastrophe such as incendiary, hurricane, or floods but through the malicious mischief or low upbringing of some maudit individuals working or hanging around as the French saying "they are clochards." The souvenirs I lost are still, yet images in my mind an Emerson radio disc player combo, that was the "bomb" at that time. The radio disc player was given to me with a disc containging a tune I can still remember "Feeling Hot! Hot! Hot!" My undergarments were also taken, all the pieces of my clothing, leaving me only with the pieces of rags I had on, also including an expensive bathrobe from Saks Fifth Avenue, given to me by a devoted girl friend, and a bottle of Courvoisier. Yes, I was feeling hot, indeed!

The vagrant who broke into my place did not know the pain I had to endure to secure these things, not knowing how much sentimental value those things held for me.

He stole my "Jockey" undergarments to cover my "culo." Perhaps it might have been the first time that he had the opportunity to carry a piece of undergarment in his life—stealing underwear I fart into, how deplorable! This act would allow him to stop swinging in the park with his "dangling" going to the cadence of a pendulum.

The mentality of these bastards is never to work in their life but wait till the time when a productive person goes to work, breaking into their home and stealing their belongings that they have worked for. These rejects of the society make the sorrow of the world.

Perhaps some of the readers might say to themselves that this man is angry. You may be right. I am not only angry, but I am also still feeling hot, so hot. I am burning and the whole fire department would not be able to extinguish my blaze. Some would also say that I do not have any compassion; compassion does not mean to encourage lawlessness. Doing nothing in your life, staying idle in your existence, is the mother of all vices. I would have had compassion for those who are handicapped and not able to help themselves, but if someone is healthy, lazy enough not to look for work and the sun shines for everyone, these people are indign to live, and their existence is purely protected by society.

Some of you would shake your heads and say that this writer has balls. Let me tell you, yes. I not only have balls but I carry them and am not afraid of castration. Only one thing I do know is that I am here to tell it just *Like It Is*.

Chapter 3

After saying a few words about my boss, let me go back to the Whitecliff ordeal. I had chosen to live at the Shangri-la because it was near the place I worked. Being dead tired after the stress of the day, I had to have a place close-by to rest. I had some sad experiences working in the field of health care. To recall, I was sharing a room with a nurse, a sloppy-looking one. One evening, we were going back and forth to the room, when I saw on the med room floor a bloody sanitary napkin. I brought it to the attention of the nurse who was sharing the room with me.

Surprisingly she said, "It is not mine."

I was astonished when the nurse with a blush on her face expelled from her mouth this embarrassing exclamation.

Ipso facto, I told her, "Miss, I am a man and I am a 100 percent man. I do not have menstruation, as you know men never have one and I am still a virgin. No one has ever played with it and I only use it to defecate. Just pick up your trash and discard it somewhere, and the next time, wear some panties, not just stick it between your legs thinking it is safe." "You are nasty."

There was a married couple sharing one room. Seemingly the man was a little impotent. Maybe his large "epiploon" made him a teaser. The couple became friendly with an African American resident. Some untoward incident occurred between the two friends. His wife raised an argument with the husband and the administrator, stating that she wanted to live alone in a single room. After many consultations and meetings, the interdisciplinary team finally agreed and accepted the wife's dalliance. Therefore, she was placed in a single room. She became happy and cheerful with a glow on her face. What had actually happened, as I was informed, that the African American resident, during the middle of the night, would sneak in her room and have a good time. At this point, the administrator got upset and wanted to charge the man with rape, but could not because the woman stated that she wanted him to copulate with her and that was her fulfilled wish. The man did not rape her but to prevent further coitus acts between the two residents, the administrator transferred the man to another facility.

At the same facility, another sexual misconduct between residents was taking place. Two men sharing a room, and one of them was retarded while the other had "family size" extension. What had happened was that the man with the "family size" got sick, complaining of pain and of not feeling well, nothing specific; a few days passed by and the pain became intolerable. The man finally made it clear to one of the staff members the cause of him having a painful extension. What had happened was that as the roommate was retarded, the man with the "giant size" extension, during the night, would enjoy himself putting his stuff in the retarded man's mouth, who chewed on it like a piece of Polish Boy.

It is said that the night shift is a dead man's shift. Some of the nurses loved to work nights so that they could sleep; therefore, no runs would be made, the residents would not have been checked, and the staff on duty had not supervised, which meant everything goes.

Let's bring to light about the time when the state surveyors would come to survey the facility. During the inspection, beds would be made with new and crispy sheets and pillowcases and new silverwares and plates would be brought out but right after the surveyors left the "new" supplies would disappear until the next year's survey.

It was not surprising that greedy and slick people own this place. Surprising was the type of food which was served to the residents. This owner went to the West Side Market twice a week at about 5:00 p.m. before the market closed to buy food at a bargain, rejects such as dehydrated veggies. The meals served to the residents: beets, mashed potatoes and blue veggies make it look like the color scheme of "old Glory".

They had a dietician; he was of the same creed as the owner and the administrator, conspiring to defraud the government, the taxpayers, and the residents.

No wonder the name of the facility had been changed. I bring this to your attention, just to blow the whistle on these types of behaviors that I had experienced, due to the fact that I had wanted to talk about them, and now what the heck! I have the opportunity to just tell it *Like It Is*.

Chapter 4

As I have previously spoken about sexual misconduct on the part of the residents, I shall now overlook the fault of the administration of some of these facilities for not providing enough help at night to make rounds routinely. I recall this Filipino nursing supervisor at night who would wind up with two keys in her hand, and if by chance the agency would send one nurse, she considers herself blessed. The residents took advantage of staffing shortage!

The administration let a young lady admitted with the diagnosis of AIDS to socialize with some of the male residents; her involvement contaminated a male resident. The male resident finally died and the female stayed busy perusing her black widowhood endeavors.

Another occasion, a male resident, who had been a truck driver, fell in love with a very pretty and frail female resident. When the relationship became stronger and stronger, the administrator decided to marry them. The marriage ceremony took place and a matrimonial room was provided to them for their honeymoon. Believe it or not, the morning after the wedding, the ambulance had to be called to take the poor lady to the hospital. Then she was transferred from the emergency room to ICU. No one could explain why marriage ended in hospitalization; the poor lady, her diagnosis had been kept confidential. Everyone kept trying to guess. We finally realized what it was: Too much! Too much!

Now we come to the DD affair. DD was an old married man who had sustained some brain injury. He became incoherent but did not forget how to touch the pie. Every evening, a heavyset female resident visited him, with his door closed. One day, a nurse, not able to resist the intense of her curiosity, knocked and opened the door. She saw DD copulating with the female. The nurse advised the female resident to go and wash up to rid herself of the pungent aroma emanating from her. This was a very difficult situation to deal with. Mr. DD. was a married man; his wife did not have the time to care for him at home during the week but took him home on weekends. I wonder if the administration ever talked to the wife about the sexual encounter of her husband and whether steps had been taken to prevent the wife from being contaminated by her husband.

Peyton place was also infected with rodents. Just stop a moment to think about it, this facility receiving mega money from the government to care for the very sick residents and not only were they short of staff, but also infested with rats. To recall, on some occasions, residents were bedfast with feeding tubes and rats would climb up the bed to bite the feeding tube, just to satisfy their satiety with milk. On one particular occasion, one nurse who had rodents' phobia saw a rat in bed with a resident. She ran out of the door and never came back to work. Many times these facts were reported to the administration. A cheap exterminating company would be sent but the result would be nil. This proved that they were greedy enough to accept residents by all means, making money, but did not have enough money to hire a good exterminator. Shame on these people!

Mr. R. for years had never walked and had always been in a wheelchair, which was self-propelled. Mr. R. reported one day that he had scratches on his legs which had since then spread and become ulcers on both lower legs. It was an ordeal for the nurse to do treatment twice a day. It took about an hour to an hour and a half to do the treatments and there was no remedy or cure for him. It was a nightmare for a nurse to have Mr. R. in her or his assignment. To recall for you, Mr. R. never walked and was wheelchair bound. One day, Dr. P. came to make a round for orders and progress notes. That day she had wanted to see Mr. R.'s ulcers. She asked the nurse to take the dressing off his legs so that she could assess the wound *de novo*.

After seeing the extent of the ulcers, Dr. P. said to Mr. R., "I can help you to feel better."

Mr. R.'s face illuminated and he said, "Doc, I will be more than glad if you could help me get better."

Dr. P. said, "You know, Mr. R., your condition is very serious. There is only one way you can get better, that is, for me to cut off both of those legs, and I can do that for you."

Mr. R. was astonished. He opened his eyes wide and said, "Hell no! Doc, I can walk!"

Mr. R., who had never walked before, got up, kicked the wheelchair aside, and started walking. It was a surprise for everyone to see Mr. R. walking. Truly, necessity is the mother of invention.

We often watch the news and often when there is a gruesome crime we hear this statement, abusing the corpse. I recall one incident when a funeral home was called to pick up a body. A signed release form was given to the attendants stating that the body was intact. The funeral home attendants attested to that because they had to sign a release form. What actually happened was that the attendants picked up the body and, while the nurse was at the window watching, the attendants dropped the body to the ground. The nurse sent a caregiver to halt the driver. She reassessed the body and asked for an incident report. Although this was not intentional, it is always recommended to pay attention to the way the residents are being transported.

Mrs. C., a 7-3 nursing supervisor, came every morning with a large thermos in her hand taking sips from the Dewar vase, leading the staff to believe that it was coffee. So selfish! She would never offer some of that good coffee she was having to anyone, not even to her close friends. One day, her coworkers and best friend asked her as to what she was drinking from her thermos.

She replied, "This is coffee to keep me energetic and awake."

This was the litany she recited every morning whenever she came to work. Some of the nurses were so curious that they asked her to share some coffee with them. Mrs. C. clearly said no!

One day, we do not know what happened. It could be that the coffee in her thermos was too strong. At that time there were no espressos, no Caribou, no Phoenix, no Starbucks. It could be that she had too many cups of that brew in her thermos. At around 11:30 a.m., Mrs. C.'s face became flushed red like a lobster and not being able to carry the load of her habit she went to a resident's bed and slept.

She was terminated on the spot. Let's go a little further; Mrs. C. was a part of the administration, birds of the same feather that existed and still exists till this day. The plantation system in the workplace will be changed eventually. Although everyone was suspicious about her habit, she was well protected by the administration due to the color of her skin. This time evidence was too tangible, the administration was not able to cover up, and they had to let her go.

I think some of you might say that I am angry about something or might have been upset about something. To make it clear to the readers, I am not upset but tired to work in a corrupt atmosphere and keep my lips sealed. I am tired with the system. Now is the time to bring these dilemmas to light and to tell it just *Like It Is*.

Chapter 5

Recall that I have talked about the administration of some of the facilities, inconveniences with their subordinates and sexual involvement with them. Now is the time to talk about some of the supervisors. It is said that birds of a feather flock together and the eagle flies alone. These following stories will open your eyes.

There was a nice-looking female nurse working under this male supervisor. Anything went, patients were neglected and employees did not do their work. One afternoon at mealtime, trays had been delivered to the floor. Three nurse's aides were on duty along with one male. Trays had been passed along to residents and the male nurse's aide was nowhere to be found to assist residents with their feeding. A female nurse's aide brought it to the attention of the supervisor that it was a normal routine for the male nurse aide to disappear at mealtimes. The nurse supervisor made a room-to-room search and this male culprit was found sleeping behind a privacy curtain. He was told to punch out and was fired on the spot. Many workers knew about this man's behavior but were afraid to speak out, worried about reprisal, or they belonged to the same click. Therefore, the residents had been neglected. It was about time to say good-bye to this neglectful caregiver.

Most of the facilities function with shortage of staff; some make deals with agencies to supply them with nurses or nurse's aides. This nurse who was sent by the agency to work as a supervisor became familiar with the facility. This nurse, once the evening shift would leave, went to bed in the basement with a male LPN. The administration knew about it but did nothing. These type of people from the administration were blinded by avarice; no wonder they were not able to live in one place and because of their greediness they had to travel all over the world and finally settle down in America. As it has been stated many times, "Only in America."

The nurse, mentioned earlier, finally disappeared. It was said that she had committed some violation and was apprehended by the police.

Another male supervisor would come to work drunk like a ceremonial goat but nothing was said to him, because he was working cheap and so the administration closed their eyes to his habit. It was also noted that some orderly would come drunk to work. The supervisor could not report it for he would be drunk himself and the fish started to get spoiled by the head. This drunk orderly had a daughter working as an LPN for the facility as well as the drunken supervisor who had his wife working there, so it was covered up all around.

The orderly's daughter, an LPN, failed to attend a patient who was having a heart attack. Instead she left the floor and stood outside talking with her boyfriend, a kitchen employee. This time it went too far. The DON did not have any excuses; she had to let her go.

The boyfriend mentioned above was a rooster in the farm, talking sweetly to most of the females on the premises. It seemed he was not able to content himself getting involved with two LPNs and also stealing checks left to be distributed to the employees the day after payday. The administration set a trap with some ink which could be detected by ultraviolet light and found out that this "Casanova" was the kitchen worker stealing checks. He was handcuffed and escorted out by police.

Shame on those women who were fighting over Mr. Goodbar, who brought shame on them. Maybe they consoled one another. One was black and the other was white, this was a *Noir et Blanc* thing!

Let me take this opportunity to give everyone this simple advice, "Never defecate where you eat." These two acts do not go together. Try to have some prestige; please do not throw the profession down the drain, at least, have some decency.

Talking about supervisors is a never-ending story. This supervisor, a mammoth looking female, had the opportunity to do her own staffing (night staffing). She told her staff, even the agency caregivers, that if they wanted to know the schedule they had to bring a dish to work at least two times a week so that they could have lunch together. It was a scheme to feed her grandchildren and herself with the food that the staff did not eat that night, which went home with her the following morning. No wonder the supervisor was that humongous and, besides all this, *"Mama Mia"* had the key to the kitchen and every night cooked some extra meals for her to take home in the morning before the dayshift crew arrived. The key to the kitchen was given to her in the event that the morning cook called off so that someone else could have breakfast ready and on time. It did not make any difference to the administration, as the people managing the place were crooks themselves. This administrator collected taxes from employees' wages and failed to report most of them to the IRS. I recall an incident about a female LPN who after working for years for this man applied for social security. She was told that she did not have enough quarters, as the man had not reported the taxes that she had collected. This same man had maintenance men on the payroll, who went to his home and performed work at the expense of the facility. There were times when a maintenance person was needed to fix a malfunction or a broken appliance and they were nowhere to be found. The residents had to remain without services until late in the afternoon, the time when the maintenance workers would punch out. This man had a heated driveway and five kitchens in his home; stealing from the taxpayers is a crime and it is about time to tell on them!

Can be there was some hanky panky between the administration and some of the physicians? To recall, one Friday evening, a call came from a hospital for a resident to be admitted on Saturday morning. The following day all pertinent information about the resident to come was sent to the house by the hospital, and the physician was also aware of the patient transfer and should have been informed about the patient arrival to the facility. That Saturday morning, one ambulance wheeled the resident on a stretcher to the room where the resident had been assigned and was put to bed by the ambulance attendants. The nurse, while taking a brief report from the attendants, found out that the patient was dead. The physician, in question, belonged to the same religion that prevents them from taking calls on Saturdays. The administrator, the DON, was also from the same culture. The ADON (assistant director of nursing) was nowhere to be found. No medical director could be contacted and no family was informed. The nurse pronounced the resident for the time being until sundown that Saturday to inform the physician of the ordeal.

It is obvious that when someone takes the Hippocratic oath to serve mankind, he should be able to care for the sick at any time; religion should not interfere with someone's duty and should not stop anyone from fulfilling his obligation in serving humanity.

Talking on the pretext that religion forbids this or that is pure bull! Accepting this excuse from a group or someone is pure tolerance as they usually say: "Only in America."

By the same token I have a heart-wrenching story to tell. We had a resident who was diabetic. This resident developed an ulcer in one of her legs. The ulcer became so bad that the only resort was to amputate the leg above the knee to save the resident's life. They scheduled to have the amputation done and after a few days of hospitalization the resident returned to the facility with special instructions. The dressing was to be changed only by the physician who performed the surgery. No one dare touch it! The doctor's orders were strictly followed and carried out. One day, while caring for the resident, the dressing from the stump fell off. To my surprise, the stump wound had been well healed and there was nothing to dress. *Ipso facto*, the director of nurses was informed and made aware about the steps to be taken to get this criminal on the spot and out of business. The DON (director of nursing) made a phone call to the physician and let him have it and no more patients were sent to him.

Considering that ambulance transportation was provided to this resident twice a week and, besides this, the physician had charged the taxpayers for his service (did only one thing "milk the cow" defrauding the system—"Doc, shame on you"), could it be that you are not the only one, but you will be paying for this abuse by a secret misery and one more time—"shame on you."

The law stipulates that a resident admitted to a home has the right to leave and come back, whenever he wanted, within a certain time period if the resident has the right mind, agreed! We understand very well that the facility is not a jail or concentration camp to hold residents against their will, but not when a resident goes out and comes back drunk like a "ceremonial goat." If this resident would stay quiet, there would not be any problem but the bacchanal partner disturbed the whole floor, preventing other residents from having a good night's sleep. Complaints to the administrator were nil; incident reports were a joke. The excuse was the administration would give the resident thirty days notice after presenting the problem to the interdisciplinary team. The thirty days never come up.

The other side of the coin was that the administration, greedy for money, did not want to let go even one resident that could have been too much money to lose. Avarice is the mother of all vices. Some of the health care providers do not have a heart. I have met the most heartless people in my life caring for the sick. I recall one poor resident with an integument different from the nursing supervisor's, sent back from the hospital with a death sentence. The resident had only a few days to live as it is usually the hospital practice to send patients to die in the home just to improve their image some way or the other.

The nurse who was a supervisor, with the same culture as the managing group, ordered the LPN to have the sick resident out of bed and then transported to a noisy place. When another nurse protested against the order, the LPN was frightened to remove the patient from the brouhaha. The DON (director of nurses), summoned to the floor, ordered the resident to be put back to bed as soon as possible so that she could rest peacefully. A dying person should be at peace with his or her family and not be disturbed by some loquacity. This above situation must be a reminder to us that we are passing on earth and that we must respect the desire of the divine by keeping it in mind; living on earth is purely a divine tolerance and everyone of us will pass. Some of us are clever enough to leave some souvenir for posterity to remind future generations that we had been there. If man knew what he was by the formation of his body, he would have been afraid to hurt his peers.

Earlier in the chapter, I mentioned a heavyset nurse supervisor's astuteness to feed her grandchildren. This nurse became so big that she was not able to move; she had a rolling gait. One night, a call came from another floor requesting her presence to assess a sick resident and make recommendations. On her way to the other floor, the supervisor fell. She automatically called for help. No one on duty was able to get her up from the floor. Finally, EMS (emergency medical service) was called. Two short emergency medical technicians arrived, tried their luck but were not able to budge her. The fire squad had to be dispatched and suddenly a tall ladder was pushed by a crane through a window; a large gait belt was placed around her waist which then pulled her up. What a calamity for this nurse! It is not that she never tried to lose weight; she had her stomach stapled, but she could not resist the temptation to gorge herself while she was hosting her voracious party at night. In life we must have conviction if we want to accomplish something. The conviction that I had was to make most of you aware of what was going on in most of the homes. I am sick and tired of this massive exploitation that is detrimental to the well-being of the nursing home population. I must tell it the way it had happened just *Like It Is*.

Chapter 6

This facility eager to have many residents supported by the state and federal government did not provide for the comfort of the residents. The technique used by the facilities was that they would delegate their social workers to contact other social workers from hospitals, have a telephonic conversation with hospital counterparts and then invite him or her for lunch. When a casual friendship would develop, the home in question would be the first priority for the patient who needed placement in a home.

The family would not know better and would agree with the social worker to send their kin to hell where care would be below standard. These kinds of facilities would accept any resident and not care where the patient goes. Most of the time there was a potentiality of spreading infection; most of the time no preparations were done for the admission. There were cases when patients would come to the room and there would be no IV pole, no oxygen tank or concentrator in the room. To recall one of a few incidents, when a resident was admitted with a breathing apparatus there were no turbine, no oxygen tank, or concentrator to connect the patient with. All of these are a result of greed. The social worker, who sent the patient to the inferno, sold the patient's comfort and well-being for a meal. The family had been duped by the so-called social worker's advice. Let me say this: Whoever wants to place one of his or her kin in the LTC facility should make sure that some type of investigation is made in terms of state survey, functioning of the facility in relation to staffing, equipment, and the overall care that a resident would be having in the facility; emphasis must be placed especially on the food (meals served to the residents). It should be taken into consideration that most of the facilities do not have a regular registered dietician. These so-called dieticians come to the facility once every one to two months and pass by like a flying nun. There is no continuity process; at times, these facilities change their registered dieticians as a snake changes its skin. Just remember that in diseases diet is very important to reestablish wellness.

Talking about food, I had mentioned before about the so-called administrator of one of the facilities who went to the West Side Market at about 5:00 p.m., the time when the market would be closing, to purchase some dehydrated veggies, which he would then serve to the residents. This is for a fact; in the name of saving money it is the best imaginable way to say. This administrator belonged to the same group, came from the same mold, and practiced the same technique before his ancestors were declared *Personae non gratae*, being chased from another land. This person would bring chicken to the facility, which perhaps had been inspected by the USDA or FDA, put them in some filthy tubs, and cut them up himself into pieces for cooking. Did I mention that the cook himself was a wine "o," a mad dog partisan, often coming to work halfway drunk? The cook also served as the maintenance man in times of need.

The assistant administrator, at mealtimes, sat in a distinguished place watching the residents while they would eat. This man would pick up whatever bread remained on the tray, to recycle them for the next meal. This man did not care about infection control. He had only one thing in his mind and that was to make money and to get wealthy at the expense of the residents and the employees. Figure out this that the man had his daughter and son-in-law on the payroll. The woman did not know bull's feet about being responsible for supplies and was never around to order or deliver them to the floors.

I remember a case about a tall man who had been admitted. This resident, upon admission, displayed some belligerent behavior, and no one was able to talk to him. When a male nurse heard about the belligerency of the new admission, he went to the room to talk to the man and find out what could have made this man so angry. After some man-to-man talk, the resident finally ventilated his feelings about his discomfort. He said that since admission he had been having problems in the bathroom. He added that each time he used the toilet, his scrotum touched the filthy water in the bowl; the man had a pendulous scrotum with respect to his height. Instantly the nurse understood the problem and that spontaneous intervention was necessary in this case. Maintenance was informed to elevate the toilet seat for the resident's comfort. The implementation took about four hours to be completed. What had happened was that there was no such apparatus at the facility and the maintenance man had to go to some other facility to fetch one and bring it.

In most of the facilities, as mentioned, the care is poor. I recall that a patient had an ulcer in one of his legs, at the ankle to be more specific. This lesion had not been treated properly. The nurse did not care about doing treatment and the resident was found to have maggots in the wound. He was sent to the hospital and one of his legs was amputated, a result of neglect. The physician in question did not care enough to check on the resident's wound. He contented himself to write notes and got paid by the state for work that was not provided or done, billing the state every month. This is what you call "milking the cow."

These homes charge the state for supplies. But what happens to the money, no one knows! This administrator's wife was an accountant. This was evidence that the man would put money in his pocket instead of promoting the comfort of the resident. Occasionally, there would be no tube to feed the residents, and if accidentally the tube would come off none would be available to replace it. The charge nurse would receive orders to wash the tube and reinsert it *de novo*, the recycle process.

If there were no briefs that could fit a particular resident, the nurse's aide would receive orders to put two small briefs on the resident. No objection would be made on the part of the employee, if any Objection is made the employee will be out of a job. What kills me most about this is that these administrators send their relatives to special nursing facilities, which accommodate their ethnocentric group, while they continue to abuse the poor people who inhabit their facilities, sucking their blood like a vampire. One of these days, they will be able to feel their ugliness just by touching their face. Don't you think it is enough?

Other nursing facilities were staffed by agencies because the boss would not be willing to pay benefits. Content with themselves, they would have nurse's aides in the evening shift to put two briefs on a resident at night, so that the nurse's aide on duty would not have to change the resident accordingly during the night. Who cares if the residents would sleep wet or develop decubitus ulcers? Closing my eyes to this would be a disgrace and I would not be able to be in peace with my consciousnesses. Oh no! I should not keep silent with all these wrongdoings; let me expose these crooks.

Sometimes a physician would be called about a resident and the physician would ask the nurse, "Is this patient mine?" He would not remember the name of the resident or any information about the resident, but he would bill the state every month on this name! The nurses themselves do not care.

This happened during rounds one morning. One of the residents told the DON (director of nursing) that "the fat nurse who worked last night spent the night sleeping on that bed." Was there any supervisor to make rounds? I am afraid not.

Some of the nurses would be most of the time chasing the orderly, looking for Mr. Goodbar, the black ink pen looking for a white Boboli to write on. What a disgrace to the profession!

I know very well that people are going to be very upset about me writing and exposing these things. I do not care a damn as to who is upset or not. I am sick and tired of these hypocrites! I must tell it *just Like It Is.*

Chapter 7

O n the subject of greediness and exploitation, let's pay some attention to the operation of a nursing facility that I worked for. The administrator was of the same creed as the ones I mentioned in the previous chapters. This man hired a dollar nurse to care for the residents. The nurse in question had been working for his wife's father since God knows when. This nurse was quite old. She would not even understand that she had to urinate, experiencing incontinency; her pants would be stained but she would pass out meds. Her mind was so messed up that she would give meds to some of the residents while the rest would do without it. The administrator knew about it, but did nothing because greed had made him blind and even incoherent. He did not care. To him it was a pleasure to exploit the system, the benefits being a heated driveway at home causing anathema to the snow. He also had a social worker to come every month signing the book regularly; the duty of social services and accounting was assigned to his wife. In this way, the buck stopped right there and the care given to the residents was inadequate.

This so-called medical director, managing the care of the resident, would be missing in action at times. To recall, there was a resident who had a tube inserted and fluid was coming from around the insertion site. The tube was maintained in place, but could not be used to feed or keep the resident hydrated. The nurse called the doctor to inform him about the resident's condition.

The doctor said, "I will speak with the DON." As it was a Saturday morning, the DON was not available. The nurse became furious and told the doctor, "Sir, the resident could become dehydrated during the weekend. This is your responsibility to make a decision about sending him to the ER. A note will be placed in the resident's record to clear the nurse from negligence." Finally the nurse said, "It is on you doctor!"

Without a second thought, the doctor gave the orders to send the resident to the ER. In this situation, the doctor was not able to take any decisions, was afraid of his shadow, and had to have the help of a so-called DON to do so.

The DON, who was weak as a flea, did not see further than her nose. She was from the Middle East and would try to psyche every nurse by asking them, "Do you love me?" This was her daily litany. She would go even further by asking a new nurse to help her straighten out the place by disciplining the nursing assistants, while she kissed them. A real mouse in a piece of cake!

In the facility, there was a nurse who was very close to the DON. This nurse did not do work at all. She would go out anytime she felt and would return at will, just passing the time, when she was supposed to be on the floor caring for the residents. Was there any conjoint relationship between the DON and that nurse? It was a puzzle to everyone.

At this same facility, there was another shocking incident which was brought to the attention of the public. The pharmacy who had some contracts to deliver the med orders was not honest. It was noted that some residents had been dead some months ago, yet the pharmacy was still send meds in their names! Was Medicaid charged for these deliveries? Medication orders were sent to the pharmacy with a special notation: "Do not send." The drugs were sent to the night tote by the pharmacy. When a nurse on duty called the pharmacy about their mistake, there would always be an excuse; it would always be an oversight. They had their way of throwing curve balls in order to dupe the benevolent attitude of the payers in the name of profit—avarice all the way.

For certain employees, drugs in the workplace were the norm. Although there was preemployment drug testing, some of the workers would get by somehow. Some of them in the workplace smoked weed and even dropped the butts or roaches on the floor. Surprisingly enough, one such day, only the housekeeper was behind the desk cleaning and when the DON confronted him with the evidence, he denied it. Drug testing was not ordered after the incident. The housekeeper continued to work and the incident became old news and started to fade away. This was a routine for most of the auxiliary staff; they would just apply for the job with the intention of recruiting new clients for the sale of their weed or narcotics. With this type of endeavor, no one was safe at the workplace.

Although the main door had a code which you had to use to get into the building, there was no security to protect the employees. Just to mention, this was the attitude of all the owners and administrators of the places mentioned in the previous chapters. These people were so greedy for money that they did not care a damn for the safety and life of their employees. Although stingy they made sure that the protocol was working.

I just want to open everyone's eyes by telling what has been, is, and will be going on in these long-term care facilities owned or managed by these types of people. No matter what type of albatross some of them will want to put around my neck, I do not care. I am here to tell it just *Like It Is*.

Chapter 8

I want the public to know that most of the time the long-term care facilities take the name of a historical icon or place to attract customers. Remember that this kind of greed has no conscience and focuses only on how to make the next dollar. The poor, the aged, the disabled, the mentally handicapped, the retarded, and the uneducated are slaves to this type of care, while society looks on in silence.

Furthermore, some of the long-term care facilities found with deficiencies by the state surveyors and the owner for some reason failed to meet their obligations toward correcting the deficiencies. The owner would then change the name of the facility passing it on to a brother or cousin or selling it to a corporation with the acquisition of shares as a clause to retain ownership.

One has to be employed in one of these facilities to find out what is going on.

Most facilities have a rehabilitation department. Some laypersons working for an agency present themselves as therapists. They just visit the residents in their rooms, do some talking, and a little exercise. This is therapy, commonly called range of motion. As these people work for an agency, everyday we see a different face; therefore, there is no continuity of care. In this way, the facility does not hire a full-time employee as they do not want to pay benefits such as vacation, personal days, and sick days. The agencies benefit from its fraudulence by charging the government an arm and a leg for services that they do not provide. Being there does not mean the work is, was, or has been done.

In these big-name facilities, perpetual neglect of the residents is the norm: neglect on the part of the administration, neglect on the part of the nurses, and neglect on the part of the nursing assistants. I shall not forget to mention verbal and mental abuse. To recall, one nurse told a resident, "My social security is paying for you to be here!"

In most facilities anything goes; let's not talk about the friendly attitude based on a channel attraction between lesbians and/or homosexuals for some.

That could explain why, in these homes, residents had been neglected even if a conscientious person reported it to the administration or his supervisor they did nothing. They are birds of a feather.

I recall a case where a so-called supervisor for some unknown reason was giving a hard time to a male nurse. It could be that she had some hidden grudge. The supervisor's daughter, who was a podiatrist at the facility, got sexually involved with a maintenance worker. Their sexual encounter in the basement was picked up by the monitor. This same man had been also involved with a social worker at the facility, who, when made aware of this love triangle, slapped the hell out of the maintenance worker; as a result the immoral bunch had to clear out. As it has been said, when there are love affairs on the job, especially in health care facilities, the residents are subjected to neglect.

A nurse would come to work every weekend. She was the eyes of the DON; with these privileges she did not have to do anything, although she had a wing to take care for herself. Practically nothing was done during the twelve hours that she had been assigned to work—"a lazy ass." To recall, Mrs. M. was a resident in this wing. She had been neglected for so long that she developed a sacrum ulcer. Although she had a treatment order, the treatment was never done. This resident's condition was so bad that one could smell the pungent odor coming out of her room as soon as you came within reach of her doorway.

Finally, Mrs. M.'s family threatened to sue and subsequently found another facility for her.

There was another resident who had gangrene in his right foot. The doctor, new to the facility and assigned to this patient, ordered ted hose for this patient. A male nurse brought it to the attention of the doctor that the resident had gangrene in the lower extremities and ted hose would contraindicate this condition. The doctor changed his mind about the ted hose and ordered some kind of treatment. The resident developed sores in the right leg and the gangrene became wet. No palliative treatment would have been beneficial to the resident. Only one thing that could be done for the resident's betterment was amputation. The nurses continued to treat the wet gangrene at their own pace, whenever they felt like it. Finally the resident got maggots in the wound. The nurse who was caring for the resident at that time wanted to keep it a secret, but another nurse wrote a note about it to make the administration aware of it. It was a real black eye to the facility. The so-called DON had to resign and nurses moved from floor to floor. Unfortunately, the resident was sent to the hospital and the leg was amputated, but the resident did not survive the surgery.

No one really knows what had happened in this case. This facility in question was like Peyton Place. A decent male nurse was not welcome. Most of the nurses were not kind to the male nurse, due to the fact that he did not have the same feathers—he was not homosexual.

This facility advertised for rehabilitation and special care. Can someone tell me who rehabilitated the residents or who gave them the special care? Let's remind them that if there is no continuity of care in the service, there is no rehabilitation and no specialized care. The campaign advertisement was just "baloney" to dupe the public.

I remember a case when a resident was admitted with a colostomy. The nurses were reluctant to give colostomy care and change the bag. Although one particular nurse objected to the practice and complained about the insufficient care that the resident was given, it was like talking to a wall. The floor manager herself was a lesbian, so she was not in a position to scold a woman. I am bringing this to the attention of the public so that they are careful about placing their relatives in any long-term care facility. My advice to you is to investigate thoroughly about the care that the facility is providing.

I am for certain that I have gotten under someone's skin. I do not care! I do not have anything to lose or to be afraid about. "I am just telling it *Like It Is.*"

Chapter 9

Let me add another chapter to the so-called high class or luxurious long-term care facilities. I tell this with a good laugh. Abuse and neglect are all over. There is this special place which hires an MD for its facility. This MD is a Dr. Kevorkian type, with the assumption, "if I let you die, I don't kill you." A family on tour was impressed by the cleanliness of the place and the type of meals the facility offered (buffet style). Without any reservation, their relatives drop in at these places. A special stipulation for receiving care from this facility is to "give me everything you have and I will take care of you until you die"—baloney!

You bring to this long-term care facility your fortune and after a few months you wind up under Medicare and Medicaid. If by chance you are sick, Dr. Kevorkian says, "Do nothing," working in agreement with the administration. Most of the time they brainwash the family not to do anything so that their personal belongings can remain in the facility even after the person is deceased.

I recall about a resident who got aspirated when a nursing assistant was feeding her. The nurse on duty sent the resident to the emergency room for evaluation *Ipso facto*. This resident was picked up by the family and brought back to the facility and the nurse was threatened with termination of employment.

In another case, a resident had pneumonia. The family, agreed upon the advice of the physician and the administration to do nothing, the resident died. Take in consideration a simple antibiotic order could have been sufficed to get rid of the infection. Was there any insurance money involved? I do not know!

On another occasion, Ms. E., who was an unmarried artist and devoted herself to painting, came to the facility with a truck full of paintings. But to great astonishment, these tableaux disappeared one by one. What happened to them, no one knows!

There was a nexus between the social worker, the payroll clerk, the activity person, and the administrator, doing their dirty work under the umbrella of good care.

Ms. Y., a very sick and dying lady, yet alert and aware of everything around her, was sitting in the corner of her room sobbing, when a nurse approached her to find out the reason for her behavior and also to give her reassurance. The resident said, "You know, Nurse, I have been working hard all of my life. The money that I had, I have paid to a company to custom-make my bed but since I have been admitted to this place I have not even seen my bed." When this nurse reiterated what the resident had said in a conference, the culprits looked at each other and said nothing. Let me tell you that these places were like plantations, white in the administration and black doing the dirty work—cleaning ass. In some of the places you could see a few dark-skinned nurses passing out the meds and most of the time these nurses were ass-kissers. The whole aspect is like a fly in a cup of milk.

If one is a little overweight, then he should forget about working in these places. On so many occasions, the question is asked whether everyone is supposed to be born skinny and stay skinny all of his or her life. What happens if you inherit genetic manifestations or endocrine conditions? If you are overweight you should not be denied the opportunity to be employed. These people should be ashamed for their bias against overweight individuals or people with an integument different from themselves.

As a matter of fact, one day a nurse asked the social worker to tell as to what should be the color of a person to be the recipient of a Medicare or Medicaid card? During a staff meeting, it was said that the door of the facility was open to all applicants and that there was a waiting list. All of the applicants were Caucasian and no dark-skinned applicants were able to walk through the door. As a result of this sensible questioning, some black applicants started to be admitted. It was not because of the time but because the place was surely and slowly reaching a decadence stage. I would also like you to know that this place was quite prejudiced; the physicians would decide to see the Caucasian residents first before seeing the black residents.

Peeling away the ugliness of the administrative staff, a nurse in a meeting told the administrative staff that they were hypocrites, due to the fact that every resident who was brought in paid the money. The state pays for everyone and there should not be any distinction in terms of caring. As I mentioned earlier in this chapter, the new residents came with all of their possessions, clothing, furniture, etc. One resident, in particular, was a buyer in one of the major clothing stores. This resident on admission brought along her fabulous pieces of designer clothing and when this resident passed on all of her clothes disappeared. Then, with great surprise, months later the activity coordinator started to dress like a Hollywood fashion model; every day she would wear a different designer piece. The administrative staff also took pieces of furniture to their homes and those who visited them at their homes said they were furnished like you would see in a gallery of Rococo. The irony of it was that whatever was not vintage, designer, and collectable was sold to the staff at a bargain price.

As I stated earlier in the chapter, Dr. K. was working with the administration to save money at the expense of the residents' well-being. In the case of Mrs. I. who had an ulcer in one of her ankles conservative treatment to the wound was not helpful. The wound became quite bad. In a staff meeting, the nurses said that they felt that the resident should go to the hospital for evaluation for possible amputation. Dr. K., under the influence of the administration, refused. Finally while a nurse's assistant was caring for the resident, she found the foot on the bed. The foot had got detached from the resident's body—in other words it fell off! The resident was sent to hospital for emergency amputation and this poor woman lived for only two years after the surgery.

As these long-term care facilities function like plantations, the administration would hire an informer to report about the employees' complaints and their dissatisfaction. Although this informer had her own assignment, she would not do her work. On so many occasions, it was found that this informer did not make the residents' beds as she should. This particular patient suffered from incontinency and usually in the morning the bed would be wet. This informer would content herself by just throwing a sheet over the bed wet with urine. The nurse aware of what was going on threatened to tell about this negligence to the head administrator. The DON, after shedding some crocodile tears, assigned the informer to another floor.

These so-called high-ranking places and corporations, having a revolving door to admit and discharge residents, also use similar tactics when they know that the state is about to survey the place. They send their residents with decubitus ulcers to Sisters' homes or to the hospital for fear of being cited for neglect or failure in providing necessary care to the residents in terms of prevention of decubitus.

Let me continue with the big brand-name facilities. Their beautiful landscaped grounds were there just to attract new applicants—"never judge an institution by its landscape!" This large beautiful facility housed the most distressful site one can imagine. In this facility, there were always friction between the caregivers and the administration. The administration's concept and attitude were so bad that the place could barely keep anyone who had some sense. It is right for me to say that the fish always starts to get spoilt by the head. In this particular place, the DON thought that she was Jupiter, and anyone who was under her should kiss her toes. This DON in question was like a yellow cab in New York, going from one long-term care facility to another, and like a swarm of bees her nursing friends follow her. These incompetent nurses under the protection of "Mama" would not do work, pressing the staff under them. They were well protected and secured, and residents would also be neglected. Any nurse who would report a wrongdoing or would want to make some change for the well-being of the residents was tagged with "a pain in the ass" stigma.

It is about time for the state to have a better control on the functioning of these facilities, for residents to have better care, and not to make the staff's duty very difficult so that they quit and be replaced by agency personnel.

I have to ask myself this question. Are they receiving kickbacks? If it is positive, posterity will tell on them and I shall continue without fear to tell it just *Like It Is*.

Chapter 10

N ow let me tell you about the religious long-term care facilities. I am going down this road to enlighten the shadowed imperceptible mind. It was a puzzle, but I had the opportunity to infiltrate the system. To tell the truth, the care given to the sick was not that good or exceptional. Some of the nurses were not even qualified to treat a horse. There was what one may call a "laissez-faire attitude" where a group of Pollacks in the name of religion were running the place sharing friendship and camaraderie to an extent such that one might think that lesbianism was involved, which might not have been a wrong impression because the religious people themselves are also of that type; a clever eye would be able to distinguish the man from the woman. Do not take me wrong but the religious people appreciated the help they received. I say help because the little pittance they gave for services was not enough for one to provide for a family; therefore, as they did not pay that much, they did not care about the services they had and the care provided to the old and religious.

The employees were from the same place with names ending with Zick, Zack, Kosky or a little group of Hispanics from Latin America, a few blacks, one from housekeeping and one an LPN, while most of the nursing assistants were black, about 95 percent. A real plantation as I mentioned in the previous chapters.

The administrative body was very prejudiced, hypocrites by nature. Yes they were! They would smile at you but behind closed doors they would call you by every name in the book. If there was an opening and a minority would come through the door looking for employment, they would say that the position was filled, but all of a sudden someone from the same bloodline would be hired. This maneuver tickles my pisiform. Let me express the embarrassment this way.

It is about that time when these people, whose ancestors had never done anything for America, had just come to the promised land for a better life and joined the crowd of oppressors to prevent the cultural, educational, and economical evolutions of the grandchildren of those people who had spent their life working in cotton fields to make America what she is today.

It is about the time when a man, no matter his origin, was considered not the pariah of the society but a true man raised to the greatness of his dignity and used to be respected by anyone no matter where he came from.

Talking about the religious long-term care facility, there are many sick residents who have not been taken care of as they should be. Consider a young lady who enters into a convent and works all of her life. She is made to believe by her superiors that she must work for the community. She goes to work everyday for about sixty to seventy years and never sees her paycheck. Most of these religious facilities have conditions that could have been taken care of since early adulthood; for example, most of them have hammer toes resulting from them wearing too narrow shoes complying with the uniform of the convent and most of them have oral problems. Either they have rotten teeth or their dentures have not been made since George Washington's time.

To recall, one Sister had been teaching the American Government for sixty years and when she was not able to work anymore she was placed in their farm waiting patiently for her end. This Sister had a kidney ailment and required dialysis. She was sent for dialysis three times a week and during that time she developed ulcers in both legs; as the care was poor, the nurses did not care enough to give necessary attention in order to promote the healing process. The Sister was neglected for so long that the ulcer became bad enough until she was placed in hospice to die with so-called dignity. The community did not want to spend money.

Recall a case, during Easter of 2009, when one of the Sisters got sick, very sick; she was not responding. The physician was called. The nurse on call was in the facility working the morning shift. This nurse on duty said that the Sister was fine, which was not correct. When the afternoon nurse brought to her attention that the Sister was dying and she did not know what to do. Therefore, the afternoon nurse took over and sent the Sister to the emergency room. The physician returned the call ninety minutes later. The situation was brought to the attention of the administrator who herself was a yo-yo and did not do anything about it. What can you expect from a neophyte? This administrator had been with the group for quite long. She had just received her nursing home administrator's license and belonged to the group that did not care about anything. One day, a nurse told another nurse, "We used to care for the residents as we care for our grandmothers. We would give meds when we wanted to and at times meds remained on the cart for two or three days and no one cared. But since you have come you have changed everything. You are a pain in the ass!" This thought process was brought to the attention of the so-called administrator who said that it was true that things were bad here and now it was getting a little bit better. During a meeting, this nurse who came on staff to bring about changes as the facility had been recently approved by the state. This nurse was brought in to help the facility comply with the state requirements. This nurse pointed out in a staff meeting that the nurses punched out two to three hours after work and stayed around without doing anything and got paid. The money could have been used to hire extra kitchen helpers to serve food instead of using housekeeping personnel, with their filthy uniforms and God knows if they ever washed their hands. Also, the money could have been spent to buy food for the residents instead of serving cold cuts every weekend. One of the Sisters stated that she would rather stay in her room on weekends as she was tired of cold cuts. The money could have been used to diversify the menu instead of serving the same meal for lunch and dinner.

In this facility, there were cases that would give chills to a concerned employee. Sister B had some problems with her electrolytes; her serum potassium was low. The physician was informed and he answered that he was not going to do anything. The so-called DON was notified about the physicians' decision. She was afraid of her shadow and did nothing. The Sister died.

Another Sister for months refused solid food but took supplements. This super nurse wrote a note to this physician asking him to discontinue all of the meds because the Sister did not want to eat, but she took her meds without difficulty and drank well. This new nurse reacted vehemently. The note never reached the physician and the Sister lived for about eight months.

The philosophy of these long-term care religious homes is to make a vow to poverty, enter the convent with the assumption that the convent will take care of you, work for your life, never see your check, and when old age knocks at the door the door would already be open to go to heaven or hell if any.

What is shocking is that the Sisters' families do not have the right to say anything. One of the Sisters stated that "her aunt passed and left her a very large sum of money." The inheritance was absorbed by the community and she never got a penny out of it.

I have been to this other long-term care religious facility for lay people; there was no difference. When you have been to one you've been to all—the same plantation mentality, different faces everyday, no continuity of care, neglect in all aspects of care, and employees not being supervised. The facilities are the same shit in different bedpans.

I recall once that at lunchtime that hamburgers were served and a resident noted some mold on the bread. The resident called the nurse and told her the bread had mold. The nurse told him that it was good and that he could eat it. The resident refused. How many times spoiled foods have been served to the residents? If the food is a donation, the expiration date is very important. And if it has not been checked, it would put the residents' health at risk.

Some people would deny it or would feel hot around the collar, because the exploitation, the neglect, the incompetence of the nursing staff, and the omnipotence of the medical body have been denounced. To make it clear, someone does need to bring to light the obscurity under which this long-term care religious facility has been functioning; thus, I do not care about what they say. I speak to inform the public and the taxpayers about what is going on in these facilities. I am just here to tell it *Like It Is*.

Chapter 11

L et me take the opportunity to touch a sensible point and it will not take a big university professor to understand what is occurring in the so-called survey by the state that the homes are subjected to every year. Usually in long-term care facilities, around the time of inspection, there is panic: the administrator is uptight, the director of nursing hysteric, nurses under pressure on the verge of having diarrhea, very concerned about their jobs; but the irony to this is that they spend a entire year fooling around, doing the wrong things, using the wrong approach, and when they know Jupiter is coming or is about to come, then consternation sets in.

To go further, some of the facilities know in advance about the date the surveyors would be visiting. There is some kind of a mole or an informer, some intuition, or some deep gut feeling which makes this long-term care facility aware in advance of the surveyors' visit. Something fishy is going on somewhere; maybe someday it will come to light and when that day comes, I will enjoy it by singing "Alleluia! God finally comes."

As it was pointed out in the previous chapters, the morning of the inspection one would see new crisp linen and new shiny silverware; residents with bad decubitus ulcers would be sent to the hospital for minor problems or to another Sister's long-term care facility to make the survey easier for them.

It was noted that the meals served were very appealing, the meal card in accordance with the residents' diet. This was for only three to four days in the surveyors' presence. At other times of the year, meal cards would not correspond with the residents' diet. The kitchen would send only a piece of paper on the tray to identify the resident, making sure he or she had something to eat. Sometimes the food looked like dog's vomit or some combination that would cut off the residents' appetite. Talking about substitution, which is for the birds, there was none; if residents refused the meal, a grilled cheese or a peanut butter sandwich was sent to the resident. Medicare and Medicaid do not pay for this kind of abuse. When surveyors are in the facility, the long-term care facility is well covered with nursing assistants but as soon as the surveyors leave, the facility becomes a decimator in terms of staffing. No wonder the lawyers are very eager to have cases of decubitus ulcers to make the facility pay. Avarice, which does not have money to hire nurse's assistant and nurses to care for the residents, will have money to pay for lawsuits. All of these things that I talk about are at the expense of the taxpayers and fatten the crooks' pockets.

I am curious to know whether there is any special treatment or preference in some long-term care facilities. I wonder how these so-called facilities pass the survey in terms of cleanliness, caring of the residents, and of building code and maintenance violations. Could it be that some of the facilities are so-called dumping grounds for the clochards and this is what most of the corporations know, using a revolving door, bouncing residents around from one facility to another Sister's facility. Only one thing that the corporations need is a so-called shameless physician as a partner to milk the cow at the expense of the taxpayers.

Where is the social worker? It seems that he or she becomes a systematist, in connivance with the heartless endeavors of the owner. Do we have to blame the social worker? I am curious to know. The public and the taxpayers are also curious to find out.

Does fate, religion, or sect play a role in the outcome of the survey? Let me point it out that if the long-term care facility belongs to a person of a particular religion or a corporation, the surveyors ease up the outcome of the verdict just to place a so-called fairness for the facility in question at the expense of the taxpayers' money.

On the contrary, if the home is doing quite bad and is not able to convince the surveyors, automatically the name of the home changes and we go back to the same vicious circle.

It is about time for the state and the public to be less tolerant and to declare adieu to all those corrupt individuals.

Even if someone agrees with me or not—I am not going to stop telling the truth—and I do not care if someone is happy or not—I wrote this piece to tell it: just *Like It Is*."

Biography

My name is Francois Degraff. I am a native of Port-au-Prince, Haiti. I was not able to speak English when I came to this country in 1965 from Port-au-Prince, Haiti. I attended the English class for foreigners in New York University. Then I went to Community College in New York in Staten Island and received a BS in science degree. I attended Brooklyn Jewish Hospital School of Nursing and became a registered professional nurse. I have worked in New York as an RN, and then at Corral Gables Hospital in Florida. I was an RN escort for the immigration department in New York for one trip to Bamaqou, Mali. I can speak Creole, French, Spanish, and English. Haunted by the desire to be a physician, I attended the Universidad Del Noreste in Tampico Mexico and then transferred to Spartan Health Science University in Texas. I passed the ECFMG in my third year of medical school. I applied for a residency but I was not successful in the first year. I continued to work as a nurse supervisor collecting data from one long-term care facility to another long-term care facility. I attended Cuyahoga Community College to become a primary instructor preparing STNA for the job market at this time.

Francois Degraff
BS, RN, MD, TTT (Train the Trainer)

In closing I would like to thank everyone who reads this book with the deepest love of my heart. I urge everyone to pass it along or to tell someone about it, perhaps your family members, your friends, especially those who have their love one in a long-term care facility or who anticipate the desire to place one of their relatives in one. This book is the product of the imperative condition of all well-being which is the truth. The truth that I practice, I tell with an invincible determination which I feel it is the right thing to do.

This book is an eye-opener for those who would have like to speak out, take action, but were afraid of retaliation and reprisal. I feel it is about the time to stand up and say something about the neglect, and abuse in the long-term care facilities residents are subjected to.

These people, I see them, I touch them, I hear them. Please let's make a difference in their lives by telling it just *Like It Is*.

www.ingramcontent.com/pod-product-compliance
Lightning Source LLC
Chambersburg PA
CBHW021929170526
45157CB00005B/2241